TABLE OF CONTENTS

Lamb and Ginger Stir Fry

Grilled Chicken Pesto Pizza

Cinnamon Sugar Cookies/Dialysis & Kidney friendly

Acorn Squash Baked with Pineapple

Alaska Baked Macaroni and Cheese

Apple & Cherry Chutney

INTRODUCTION

Eating well is an important part of your treatment and can help you feel better.

A new diet is essential part to your treatment process. Not only will it help you feel better, it can also help you avoid complications of your renal disease such as fluid overload, high blood potassium, bone disease, and weight loss. Because every individual is different and their needs unique, the following dietary advice should be given depending on a number of factors and discussion with your renal dietician. These factors include: stage of your renal disease, type of treatment you are on, laboratory results, and presence of other medical conditions.

Kidney function is essential for removing the waste material from food that you eat. The kidneys excrete a dietary protein called urea, as well as sodium, potassium, and phosphate. These substances can build up in the body if kidney function is impaired. Following a strict diet can lessen this accumulation and its effects.

Hemodialysis Patients should monitor and limit their intake of the following:

• Potassium

• Phosphate

• Sodium

- Fluids

Controlling Your Phosphorus

Phosphorus is a mineral that healthy kidneys get rid of in the urine. In kidneys that are failing, phosphorus builds up in the blood and may cause many problems including muscle aches and pains, brittle, easily broken bones, calcification of the heart, skin, joints, and blood vessels. To keep your phosphorus levels in check, consider the following tips:

LIMIT HIGH PHOSPHORUS FOODS SUCH AS:

• Meats, poultry, dairy and fish (you should have 1 serving of 7-8 ounces)

• Milk and other dairy products like cheese (you should have one 4 oz. serving)

Avoid high phosphorus foods such as:

• Lima Beans, Black Beans, Red Beans, Black-eyed Peas, White Beans, and Garbanzo Beans

• Dark, whole or unrefined grains

• Refrigerator doughs like Pillsbury

• Dried vegetables and fruits

• Chocolate

• Dark colored sodas

Don't forget to take your phosphate binders with meals and snacks.

• Your doctor will prescribe a medication called a phosphate binder which will be some type of polymer gel or calcium medication. You need to take your phosphate binder as prescribed by your doctor. Often you will take a phosphate binder with every meal and snack.

Usually your diet is limited to 1000 mg of phosphorus per day.

Controlling Your Potassium

Potassium is an element that is necessary for the body to keep a normal water balance between the cells and body fluids. All foods contain some potassium, but some contain larger amounts.

Normal kidney function will remove potassium through urination. Kidneys that are not functioning properly cannot remove the potassium in the urine, so it builds up in the blood. This can be very dangerous to your heart. High potassium can cause irregular heart beats and can even cause the heart to stop if the potassium levels get to high.

Typically, there are no symptoms for someone with a high potassium level. If you are concerned about your potassium level, check with your doctor, and follow the tips below.

Usually a renal patient's diet should be limited to 2000 mg of potassium each day.

THE FOLLOWING FOODS ARE HIGH IN POTASSIUM:

- Bananas
- Avocado
- Oranges
- Orange Juice
- Prunes
- Prune Juice
- Tomatoes
- Tomato Juice
- Tomato Sauce
- Cantaloupe
- Tomato Puree
- Honeydew Melon
- Nuts
- Papaya
- Chocolate

- Red Beans

- Milk

- White Beans

- Lima Beans

- Garbanzo Beans

- Black Beans

- Lentils

- Split peas

- Baked Beans

Controlling Your Sodium

Sodium, or sodium chloride, is an element that is used by all living creatures to regulate the water content in the body. Usually a sodium restriction comes in the form of "No Added Salt." This is necessary because a greater intake of sodium will result in poorly controlled blood pressure and excessive thirst which can lead to difficulty adhering to the fluid restrictions in your diet.

To limit your sodium, you should:

- Avoid table salt and any seasonings that end with the word "salt"

- Avoid salt substitutes (they contain potassium)

- Avoid salty meats such as bacon, ham, sausage, hot dogs, lunch meats, canned meats, or bologna

- Avoid salty snacks such as cheese curls, salted crackers, nuts, and chips

- Avoid canned soups, frozen dinners, and instant noodles

• Avoid bottled sauces, pickles, olives, and MSG

Controlling Your Protein

Protein is important to aid in growth and maintenance of body tissue. Protein also plays a role in fighting infection, healing of wounds, and provides a source of energy to the body.

• You should make sure to eat 7-8 ounces of protein every day. Foods that are high in protein include beef, pork, veal, chicken, turkey, fish, seafood, and eggs.

• 1 egg is equal to 1 ounce of protein, and three ounces of protein is comparable to the size of a deck of cards.

Controlling Your Fluid Intake

People on dialysis often have decreased urine output, so increased fluid in the body can put unnecessary pressure on the person's heart and lungs.

• A fluid allowance for individual patients is calculated on the basis of 'urine plus 500ml.' The 500 ml covers the loss of fluids through the skin and lungs.

• Most patients will not urinate as much once they begin Hemodialysis.

• Those who produce a lot of urine may be able to drink more than those who do not produce urine.

• Between each dialysis treatment, patients are expected to gain a little weight due to the water content in foods (fruits and vegetables).

• The amount of fluid in a typical day's meal (excluding fluids such as water, tea, etc.) is at least 500 ml and therefore expected daily weight gain is between 0.4 – 0.5kg.

- To control fluid intake, patients should:

➤ Not drink more than what your doctor orders (usually 4 cups of fluid each day)

➤ Count all foods that will melt at room temperature (Jell-O®, popsicles, and fruit ices).

RECIPES

Golden Potato Croquettes

Prep Time: 20 minutes

Cook Time: 20 minutes

Serving: 2

Ingredients

• low potassium potatoes cooked as per low potassium recipe - 400g (1lb) mashed

• unsalted butter - 25g (1oz)

• milk - ½ tablespoon

• salt - ¼ teaspoon

• black pepper - ¼ teaspoon

• egg - ½ medium sized, beaten

• fresh white breadcrumbs - 90g (3½ oz)

• olive oil - for frying (approx 3 tbsp)

Instructions

• Cook the potatoes as per the recipe for Low Potassium Potatoes

• Place the cooked low potassium potatoes, butter, milk and seasoning into a bowl and mash

- Shape the croquette with your hand and dip in the beaten egg.

- Roll each croquette in the breadcrumbs

- Heat a little olive oil in a frying pan and when hot, place the croquettes in a few at a time, making sure you have sufficient room turn them easily.

- Fry on all sides until crisp and golden. Keep warm until all are ready.

Nutrition Facts (Per Portion)

- Calories: 570kcal

- Carbohydrate: 70g

- Fat: 30g

- Protein: 10g

- Salt : 1.2g

- Sugar: 4g

- Potassium: 10mmol / 398mg

- Phosphate: 5 mmol / 157mg

CHICKEN FAJITAS

Portions: 4

Serving Size: 2 fajitas

Ingredients

- 8 flour tortillas, 6" size

- 1/4 cup green pepper

- 1/4 cup red pepper

- 1/2 cup onion

- 1/2 cup cilantro

- 2 tablespoons canola oil

- 12 ounces boneless chicken breasts

- 1/4 teaspoon black pepper

- 2 teaspoons chili powder

- 1/2 teaspoons cumin

- 2 tablespoons lemon juice

Preparation

- Preheat oven to 300° F. Wrap tortillas in foil; heat in oven for 10 minutes.

- Chop the peppers, onion and cilantro. Cut chicken breasts into 1" strips.

• Place oil in nonstick frying pan over medium heat; add chicken, seasonings and lemon juice. Cook for 3 to 5 minutes.

• Add peppers and onion to frying pan; cook for 3 to 5 minutes more or until chicken is no longer pink and juice run clear. Add cilantro to chicken mixture.

• Divide chicken mixture between tortillas; fold tortillas over.

Helpful hints

• For a lower protein diet decrease chicken portion to match your meal plan.

Nutrients per serving

• Calories 343

• Protein 24 g

• Carbohydrates 33 g

• Fat 13 g

• Cholesterol 53 mg

• Sodium 281 mg

• Potassium 331 mg

• Phosphorus 196 mg

• Calcium 23 mg

• Fiber 2.0 g

Renal and renal diabetic food choices:

• 3 meat

• 2 starch

- 1 vegetable, low potassium

RENAL-FRIENDLY HOMEMADE SAUSAGE PATTIES

Ready In: 35mins

Serves: 16

Ingredients

- ½ cup onion, finely chopped
- 2 tablespoons olive oil
- 2 teaspoons dried sage
- 1 teaspoon fresh ground black pepper
- 1 tablespoon sugar or 1 tablespoon brown sugar
- ⅛ teaspoon crushed red pepper flakes
- 1 pinch ground cloves
- 1 teaspoon fresh thyme, finely chopped
- 1 large egg yolk
- 2 lbs ground lean pork

Directions

- Cook onion in the olive oil over moderately low heat.

• Stir occasionally until onions begin to soften and brown.

• 8-10 minutes.

• Cool for 10 minutes.

• In a small bowl, combine the sage, pepper (red and black), sugar, cloves and thyme.

• Place the egg yolk, pork, and reserved onion in a large bowl and then add the mixed spices.

• Mix well.

• Form into 16 patties, 2 ounces each.

• Pan fry the patties in a large skillet over medium high heat for 5 minutes on each side or until the internal temperature reaches 160 degrees.

LEACHED MASHED POTATOES WITH ROASTED GARLIC

Servings: 4

Ingredients

• 2 large potatoes peeled and diced

• 1 head garlic

• 1 Tbsp olive oil

• 1 Tbsp butter

• 1/4 cup milk

• black pepper to taste

• chives for garnish

• parsley for garnish

Instructions

• Preheat oven to 400 degrees F. Place potato in pot and fill with cool water and bring to a boil.

• Meanwhile, cut the top of the garlic head so that the cloves are exposed and drizzle with olive oil. Wrap in aluminum foil and place in oven. Roast for 30 minutes, until softened and golden brown.

• Once the potatoes have come to a boil, pour out the water and add new water to cover the potatoes. Bring to a boil again, then continue to cook until potatoes are soft. Drain completely. Add butter, milk, and desired amount of garlic. You can use about half of the head of garlic.

• Mash the potatoes. Season with pepper to taste. Garnish with chives or parsley.

Nutrition Facts

• Carbohydrates: 36g

• Protein: 5g

• Fat: 7g

• Sodium: 42mg

• Potassium: 818mg

• Fiber: 3g

TANDOORI BITES

Prep Time: 30 minutes

Cook Time: 15 minutes

Serving: 4

Ingredients

• lean beef chopped into chunks - 225g / 9oz

• curry powder - 1 tablespoon

• lemon juice - 1 tablespoon

• cream - 3 tablespoons

• freshly chopped mint - 1 tablespoon

Instructions

• Mix all the marinade ingredients together in a bowl. Add the chopped meat, mix thoroughly, cover and refrigerate.

• Marinade for at least 30 min (max 4 hours)

• Remove the meat and thread onto metal skewers.

• Cook under a preheated grill or barbeque for approximately 15 minutes, turning occasionally.

Nutrition Facts (Per Portion)

• Calories: 118 kcal

• Carbohydrate Content: 1g

- Fat Content: 7g

- Protein Content: 13g

- Salt : 0.1g

- Sugar Content: 0.4g

- Potassium: 5.6mmol / 219mg

- Phosphate: 3.8mmol / 117mg

Vegan Lettuce Wrap

Total Time: 40 min

Prep Time: 15 min

Cook Time: 25 min

Servings: 2 (2 wraps each)

Ingredients

- ¼ cup white rice, dry

- 1 cup cauliflower

- 1 clove of garlic

- 1 teaspoon ginger, fresh

- 2 teaspoons brown sugar

- 2 tablespoons peanut butter

- 1 tablespoon reduced sodium soy sauce

- 1 tablespoon sesame oil

- 2 tablespoons rice vinegar

- ¼ pound (4 ounces) extra firm tofu

- 1 tablespoon canola oil

- ½ cup carrots, shredded or grated

- 4 medium leaves bibb or butter lettuce

Preparation

- Pre-heat oven to 400F.

- Cook rice according to package directions, omitting any salt or butter.

- Chop the cauliflower into very small pieces, to a rice-like consistency.

- Mince the garlic and ginger. Blend the garlic, ginger, brown sugar, peanut butter, soy sauce, sesame oil, and rice vinegar in a small blender. Set aside.

- Pat the tofu dry with a paper towel. Cut into bite sizes pieces. Toss with canola oil and bake for 20 minutes at 400F, flipping halfway through.

- When the rice is done cooking, turn off the heat and mix in the cauliflower.

- When the tofu is done cooking, scoop it into a bowl and mix with the peanut butter sauce.

- Put the lettuce leaves on a plate. Fill with rice/cauliflower mixture, then shredded carrots, then tofu. Drizzle any leftover sauce on top.

Ingredient Variation and Substitutions:

- Use pre "riced" cauliflower if you can find it. Measure out

2/3 cup for this recipe.

• Other types of lettuce can be substituted, but bibb and butter lettuce fold the best.

• Top with crushed red pepper if you like it hot.

Cooking and Serving Tips:

• The more you pat-dry the tofu, the crispier it will get when it cooks.

Nutrition Highlights (Per Serving)

• 410 calories

• 26g fat

• 34g carbs

• 14g protein

SHEPHERD'S PIE WITH CAULIFLOWER AND BUTTERNUT SQUASH MASH

Paleo, Keto and Whole30-friendly, this shepherd's pie satisfies your taste buds and your eating plan.

Prep: 10 Min

Active: 20 Min

Passive: 45 Min

Serves: 2-4 Servings

Ingredients

Meat and Veggie Filling:

- 1 lb. PRE ground beef

- 1 ½ cups rainbow carrots (diced)

- 1 ½ cups frozen green beans (chopped)

- 1 large shallot (sliced)

- 2 garlic cloves (minced)

- 2 tbsp. ghee or butter

- ½ tbsp. tomato paste

- ½ tbsp. coconut aminos

- ½ tsp. salt

- ½ tsp. black pepper

- ½ tsp. ground rosemary

- ½ tsp. thyme

Cauliflower and Butternut Squash Mash Topping:

- 2 cups butternut squash (peeled and diced)

- 2 cups cauliflower florets

- 1 tbsp. ghee or butter

- 2 tbsp. coconut cream

- ¼ tsp. salt

- ¼ pepper

Instructions

- Fill large saucepan with water and bring to a boil. Add in cauliflower florets and diced butternut squash, then reduce to a simmer. Cook for about fifteen minutes, or until soft.

- Drain cauliflower and squash, then add to food processor or use immersion blender. Add one tablespoon of ghee (or butter), two tablespoons of coconut cream, salt, and pepper. Blend until smooth and set aside in a bowl.

- Add one tablespoon of ghee (or butter) to large pan on medium heat, and mix in half of shallots and crushed garlic. Cook for about 1-2 minutes, then add ground beef.

• Season with one half teaspoon of salt and pepper and break beef into small pieces. Cook until browned (about 5-7 minutes), then place in bowl and set aside. Drain grease from pan.

• In same pan, cook veggies. Add one tablespoon of ghee (or butter) to pan on medium heat, and incorporate remaining shallots and garlic. Cook for 1-2 minutes, and then add diced carrots and chopped green beans. Sprinkle salt and pepper. Add half teaspoon of rosemary and thyme, and cook for 5-7 minutes until carrots are slightly soft.

• Once veggies are cooked, add ground beef back to the pan. Add half tablespoon of tomato paste and coconut aminos. Stir well until fully incorporated. Then, remove from pan and place in baking dish.

• Add cauliflower and butternut squash mash over top of meat and veggie filling. Preheat oven to 375F. Bake for about thirty minutes, or until edges are golden. Let sit for 5-10 minutes.

• Enjoy!

GARLIC MASHED POTATOES

Portions: 4

Serving Size: 1/2 cup

Ingredients

- 2 medium potatoes

- 2 garlic cloves

- 1/4 cup butter

- 1/4 cup 1% low fat milk

Preparation

- Peel and slice the potatoes into small pieces.Double-boil to reduce potassium if you are on a low potassium diet. (See helpful hints.)

- Boil potatoes and garlic over medium heat until soft.

- Drain off cooking water.

- Whip potatoes and garlic with beater, slowly adding butter and milk until whipped smooth.

Helpful hints

- Double the garlic for a stronger garlic flavor.

• Potatoes are very high in potassium but you can remove part of the potassium by using one of these methods:

• Double boil method: Peel and small dice potatoes. Place in a large pot of water and bring to a boil. Drain the water and add fresh water to the pot. Bring to a boil, cook for 10 minutes then drain and prepare as desired.

• Leaching method: Peel and dice potatoes. Place in a large pot of warm tap water and soak for 2 to 4 hours. Drain and cook as desired.

• Leached potatoes can be blanched and frozen in batches. To blanch vegetables, add to boiling water for one minute, remove and rinse in cold water before freezing.

• Potassium content taken from reference values for double-boiling small peeled and diced potatoes.

Nutrients Per Serving

• Calories 185

• Protein 2 g

• Carbohydrates 15 g

• Fat 13 g

• Cholesterol 0 mg

• Sodium 103 mg

• Potassium 205* mg

• Phosphorus 65 mg

• Calcium 35 mg

• Fiber 0.7 g

Renal and renal diabetic food choices:

- 1/2 starch

- 1 vegetable, medium potassium

- 2 fat

- Carbohydrate choices 1

APPLE CINNAMON FRENCH TOAST STRATA

Portions: 12

Serving Size: 3" x 3" square

Ingredients

• 1 pound loaf cinnamon raisin bread

• 8 ounces cream cheese

• 1-1/2 medium apples

• 6 tablespoons unsalted butter

• 1 teaspoon ground cinnamon

• 8 large eggs

• 1-1/4 cup half & half creamer

• 1-1/4 cup almond milk, unsweetened, original

• 1/4 cup pancake syrup

Preparation

• Dice the bread and cream cheese into cubes. Peel and dice the apples. Melt the butter.

• Coat a 9" x 13" baking dish with nonstick cooking spray. Arrange 1/2 of the cubed bread in the bottom of the dish. Sprinkle the cream cheese cubes evenly over the bread and top with the apples. Sprinkle cinnamon over the apples and top with remaining bread.

• In a large bowl, beat the eggs with the half & half creamer, almond milk, melted butter and pancake syrup. Pour the mixture over the bread. Cover baking dish with plastic wrap and press down so that all the pieces are soaked. Refrigerate at least 2 hours or overnight

• Preheat oven to 325° F.

• Bake the strata for 50 minutes, then let stand 10 minutes before serving. Cut evenly into squares for 12 servings.

• Top with pancake syrup, sugar-free syrup, jam or cinnamon/raspberry applesauce, if desired.

Renal and renal diabetic food choices:

• 1 meat

• 1-1/2 starch

• 1/2 fruit

• 2 fat

• Carbohydrate choices 2

Nutrients Facts Per Serving

• Calories 324

• Protein 9 g

• Carbohydrates 27 g

• Fat 20 g

- Cholesterol 170 mg

- Sodium 280 mg

- Potassium 224 mg

- Phosphorus 150 mg

- Calcium 116 mg

- Fiber 1.8 g

LOW POTASSIUM FRIED POTATOES

Serves: 4

Prep: 5 Min

Cook: 15 Min

Ingredients

- 2 medium potatoes, peeled

- 1/2 c canola oil

- 1/4 tsp ground cumin

- 1/4 tsp paprika

- 1/8 tsp ground white pepper

- 8 tsp catsup

- 1/2 c onions, small white

Preparation

- Slice each potato into 16 pieces approximately 4" x 1/2" each.

- Soak cut potatoes in a gallon of tap water for 2 to 4 hours to reduce potassium. Drain and pat dry with paper towels.

- Heat oil over medium heat in a skillet. Add potatoes to

hot oil and cook for 10 to 12 minutes until golden brown.

• Remove fried potatoes to a paper towel to absorb extra oil.

• Combine cumin, paprika and white pepper in a small dish or shaker. Sprinkle over hot potatoes and toss.

• Serve 8 fries with 2 teaspoons ketchup.

Nutrients Serving size: 8 pieces (4" x 1/2" each)

• Calories: 156

• Protein: 2 g

• Carbohydrate: 21 g

• Fat: 7 g

• Cholesterol: 0 mg

• Sodium: 134 mg

• Potassium: 181 mg

• Phosphorus: 54 mg

• Calcium: 10 mg

• Fiber: 1.7 g

Renal and renal diabetic food choices:

• 1 starch

• 1 vegetable, medium potassium

• 1 fat

Carbohydrate choices

• 1

Helpful hints

• Soaking potatoes is very important to reduce potassium. Potatoes are very high in potassium. Consuming high potassium foods in advanced kidney disease may cause high blood potassium levels, muscle weakness and heart failure.

• Dry potatoes well before adding to hot oil.

• If no salt added ketchup is substituted for regular ketchup sodium will be reduced to 7 milligrams per serving. (Avoid brands containing potassium chloride).

Lamb Koftas with Tzatziki Sauce

Prep Time: 60 minutes

Cook Time: 30 minutes

Serving: 4

Ingredients

• lamb - 500g / 20oz minced

• onion - 1 medium (150g / 6oz), finely chopped

• garlic - 2 cloves, crushed

• fresh coriander - 1 tablespoons of finely chopped

• olive oil - 1 tablespoon

• black pepper - 1 level teaspoon, freshly ground

• pitta bread - 4 pockets

Tzatziki Sauce:

- sour cream - 300mls / 10 fluid ounces

- cucumber - ½, grated

- garlic - 1 clove, crushed

- mint - 2 tablespoon, finely chopped

Fresh Salad:

- lettuce - 3 leaves

- cucumber - 2 slices

- tomato - 1 slice

- red onion - 1 slice

Instructions

- To make the lamb koftas, put all the ingredients into a large bowl and mix well.

- Season with freshly ground black pepper.

- Shape the mixture into 16 balls, each about the size of a golf ball.

- Cover the lamb koftas with clingfilm and place in the fridge to set for 1 hour.

- Add 1 tablespoon of olive oil to a frying pan and place over a medium heat.

- Brown the lamb koftas on all sides then allow to cook for a further 6-8 minutes.

- While the lamb is cooking make the tzatziki sauce. Place all the ingredients in a bowl and stir to combine. Allow the sauce to chill in the fridge prior to serving.

- Ensure lamb koftas are cooked thoroughly prior to serving.

• Serve the lamb koftas in pitta bread pockets, with the tzatziki sauce and fresh salad.

• Ensure all salad vegetables are thoroughly washed prior to serving.

Nutrition Facts (Per Portion)

• Calories: 585kcal

• Fat Content: 32g

• Protein Content: 29g

• Salt : 1g

• Sugar Content: 10g

• Potassium: 769mg/ 20mmol

• Phosphate: 12mmol / 371mg

CHICKEN AND GNOCCHI DUMPLINGS

Classic comfort food made kidney-friendly. This hearty, yet quick and easy chicken soup uses fresh gnocchi as the dumplings.

Serves: 10 (1 serving = 1 cup portion)

Ingredients

• 2 pounds chicken breast

• 1 pound gnocchi (store bought)

• ¼ cup grape seed or light olive oil

• 1 tablespoon Better Than Bouillon® Chicken Base (low sodium)

• 6 cups reduced-sodium chicken stock

• ½ cup fresh celery, finely diced

• ½ cup fresh onions, finely diced

• ½ cup fresh carrots, finely diced

• ¼ cup fresh parsley, chopped

• 1 teaspoon black pepper

- 1 teaspoon Italian seasoning

Directions

- Place stockpot on stove, add oil and set to high heat.

- Place chicken in hot oil and brown on all sides until golden brown.

- Add celery, carrots and onions and continue to cook with chicken until translucent. Add chicken stock and let cook on high heat for 20–30 minutes.

- Reduce heat and add chicken bouillon, black pepper and Italian seasoning; then stir. Add gnocchi and cook for 15 minutes, stirring constantly.

- Remove from stove, add parsley and serve.

Tip

- Save extra soup for an easy leftover meal. It can be frozen until ready to defrost, heat and serve.

Tortilla Beef Rollups

Serving Size: 1 rollup or 4 pieces

Ingredients

- 2 flour tortilla, 6" size

- 2 tablespoons whipped cream cheese

- 5 ounces roast beef, cooked

- 1/4 cup red onion, chopped

- 1/4 sweet bell pepper (red, yellow or green), cut in strips

- 8 cucumber slices

- 2 romaine lettuce leaves

- 1 teaspoon herb seasoning blend

Instruction

- Spread cream cheese over tortillas.

- Divide ingredients in half to make two torillas. Layer each tortilla with roast beef, red onion, pepper strips, cucumbers and lettuce.

- Sprinkle with Mrs. Dash® herb seasoning blend.

- Roll up like a jellyroll.

- Slice each tortilla into 4 pieces, or serve whole.

Renal and renal diabetic food choices

- vegetable, low potassium

- 3 meat

- 1 starch

- Carbohydrate choices 1

Nutrients Facts

- Calories 258

- Protein 24 g

- Carbohydrates 18 g

- Fat 10 g

- Cholesterol 72 mg

- Sodium 279 mg

- Potassium 448 mg
- Phosphorus 253 mg
- Calcium 59 mg
- Fiber 1.6 g

GOLDEN POTATO CROQUETTES

Prep Time: 20 minutes

Cook Time: 20 minutes

Serving: 2

Ingredients

- low potassium potatoes cooked as per low potassium recipe - 400g (1lb) mashed
- unsalted butter - 25g (1oz)
- milk - ½ tablespoon
- salt - ¼ teaspoon
- black pepper - ¼ teaspoon
- egg - ½ medium sized, beaten
- fresh white breadcrumbs - 90g (3½ oz)
- olive oil - for frying (approx 3 tbsp)

Instructions

- Cook the potatoes as per the recipe for Low Potassium Potatoes
- Place the cooked low potassium potatoes, butter, milk

and seasoning into a bowl and mash

• Shape the croquette with your hand and dip in the beaten egg.

• Roll each croquette in the breadcrumbs

• Heat a little olive oil in a frying pan and when hot, place the croquettes in a few at a time, making sure you have sufficient room turn them easily.

• Fry on all sides until crisp and golden. Keep warm until all are ready.

Nutrition Facts (Per Portion)

• Calories: 570kcal

• Carbohydrate: 70g

• Fat: 30g

• Protein: 10g

• Salt : 1.2g

• Sugar: 4g

• Potassium: 10mmol / 398mg

• Phosphate: 5 mmol / 157mg

Low Salt Gravy

Prep Time: 10 minutes

Cook Time: 10 minutes

Serving: N/A

Ingredients

• meat juices

• gravy browning - (a product that will add colour and flavour)

• cornflour

• herbs, spices, onions - for flavouring

Instructions

• Allow the meat juices to cool and skim off the fat

• Thicken with cornflour

• Add gravy browning until the gravy is the colour you want

• Add flavourings as you wish

• Don't use stock cubes or gravy mixes

• Use gravy sparingly and include as part of your fluid allowance

Roast Crown of Turkey with Sage and Onion Stuffing

Roast Crown of Turkey with Sage and Onion Stuffing

Serving: 8

Ingredients

• Ready - prepared Turkey Crown - 4.5kg (10lb)

• Butter, at room temperature - 75g (3 oz)

- 1 garlic clove, crushed

- Finely grated zest of 1 orange

- Fresh flat leaf parsley, chopped - 1 level tbsp

- Fresh thyme, chopped - 1 level tsp

For the Stuffing:

- Butter - 75g (3oz)

- 1 small onion, diced

- Fresh sage, chopped - 1 level tsp

- fresh white breadcrumbs - 175g (6oz)

- Freshly ground black pepper - pinch (1/4 level teaspoon)

Instructions

- Preheat the oven to 190 degrees celcius / 375 degrees fahrenheit / Gas 5.

- To make the stuffing, heat a frying pan and melt the butter.

- Add the onion and sage and cook for a few minutes, until softened but not coloured.

- Stir in the breadcrumbs, mixing well to combine.

- Season with freshly ground black pepper.

- Wrap the stuffing in buttered tinfoil and mould into a large sausage shape.

- This can be cooked in the oven for 25 - 30 minutes.

- Next, prepare the Turkey Crown.

- Cream the butter in a bowl until very soft and then add

the crushed garlic, orange rind, parsley and thyme.

• Beat well, until thoroughly blended.

• Gently loosen the neck flap away from the breast and pack the flavoured butter right under the skin - this is best done using gloves on your hands.

• Rub well into the flesh of the turkey, then re-cover the skin and secure with a small skewer.

• Place the turkey crown in the oven and calculate your time. You should allow 20 minutes per 450g (1lb) plus 20 minutes, so a joint this size should take 3 hours and 40 minutes.

• Cover loosely the foil and remove this about 40 minutes before the end of cooking time.

• The turkey crown will cook much quicker than a whole turkey, so make sure to keep basting.

• To check if the turkey is cooked, pierce a fine skewer into the chest part of the crown - the juices should run clear.

• When cooked, cover with foil to rest and keep warm.

• To serve, carve the turkey crown into slices and arrange 125g (5 oz) on warmed plates with the cooked stuffing.

LOW POTASSIUM VEGETABLES

Prep Time: 10 minutes

Cook Time: 20 minutes

Serving: N/A

Ingredients

• Root Vegetables - As many as required

Instructions

• Choose root vegetables that are naturally lower in potassium. Your Kidney (Renal) Dietitian can provide you with a list of suitable vegetables.

• Peel the vegetables

• Chop into small pieces and place into a pot for boiling. The pot must be large enough to hold the required volume of water.

• Cover the vegetable with four times their volume in fresh boiling water.

• Place a lid onto the pot and put onto a high heat.

• Bring the water to the boil and then reduce the heat and simmer until cooked.

• Drain and measure out your vegetable allowance. Your Kidney (Renal) Dietitian can help to set and explain about your daily vegetable allowance.

Blue Cheese Spread with Melba Toast

Prep Time: 10 minutes

Cook Time: 10 minutes

Serving: 4 People

Ingredients

• Cream Cheese - 150g (5 oz)

• Stilton - 25g (1oz)

• ground black pepper - ¼ teaspoon

• brown sliced pan - 2 slices

Instructions

• In a mixing bowl beat the two cheeses and pepper together until well blended.

• Remove crusts from bread and toast lightly.

• Using a bread knife carefully split the slices through the middle and toast the uncooked surfaces under a hot grill until crisp and brown.

• Spread the cheese mix onto the melba toast and serve

Nutrition Facts (Per Portion)

• Calories: 233kcal

- Carbohydrate: 7.6g

- Fat: 21g

- Protein: 4.6g

- Salt : 0.6g

- Sugar: 0.5g

- Potassium: 3mmol / 114mg

- Phosphate: 3mmol/96mg

Salmon and Chive Pate

Prep Time: 5 minutes

Cook Time: 10 minutes

Serving: 8

Ingredients

- tin salmon - 200 g (8oz) tin salmon with no bones, rinsed & drained

- cream cheese - 100 g (4 oz) cream cheese, softened

- mayonnaise - 5 heaped tablespoons

- lemon juice - 2 tablespoons

- margarine/ butter - 50 g (2 oz) melted

- fresh chives - 2 tablespoons, chopped

Instructions

- Blend the salmon, cream cheese, mayonnaise and juice until well combined.

• Gradually add the melted margarine whilst the blender is still running and blend until smooth.

• Stir in the chives

• Pour the mixture into small ramekins and refrigerate until set

• Can be served with crackers or toast.

Nutrition Facts (Per Portion)

• Calories: 282kcal

• Carbohydrate: 0.5g

• Fat Content: 28g

• Protein: 6.5g

• Salt : 0.7g

• Sugar: 0.4g

• Potassium: 2.4mmol / 94mg

• Phosphate: 63mg / 2 mmol

CRÈME BRULE

Prep Time: 30 minutes

Serving: 2

Ingredients

• pineapple slices - 2 tinned, (80g / 3oz)

• carton of double cream - 142ml (5 fluid ounces)

• small egg - 1

• castor sugar - 50g (2oz)

• Vanilla essence or brandy - ½ teaspoon

Instructions

• Preheat the oven to 150°C (Gas Mark 2).

• Pat the pineapple dry with some kitchen paper, coarsely chop and place in the bottom of 2 greased ramekin dishes (approx 8-9cm diameter).

• Heat the cream gently until it bubbles around the edge, but do not boil.

• Add half the sugar to the egg in a mixing bowl and whisk until well blended. Gradually whisk in the cream, then stir in the vanilla essence or brandy.

• Pour the mixture over the pineapple to 1cm below the rim of the dish.

• Place the ramekins in a shallow roasting dish filled with boiling water to a depth of 3cm or ¾ the depth of the ramekin.

• Bake in the oven for 25-30 minutes or until the custard is set. Remove and cool. Chill for a minimum of 1 hour or overnight.

• Preheat the grill to the hottest setting.

• Sprinkle the remaining sugar evenly over the top of the custard. Grill until brown and bubbling. Cool and chill for 1 hour before serving.

Nutrition facts (per portion)

• Calories: 504kcal

• Carbohydrate: 31 g

• Fat: 41g

• Protein: 4.4g

• Salt : 0.1g

• Sugar: 31g

• Potassium: 3.7mmol / 143.5mg

• Phosphate: 3mmol / 91 mg

Apple Crumble

Prep Time: 10 minutes

Cook Time: 50 minutes

Serving: 4

Ingredients

• cooking apples - 450 g (18 oz) peeled cored and thinly sliced

• brown sugar - 75 g (3 oz)

• plain flour - 100 g (4 oz)

• rolled oats - 75 g (3 oz)

• ground cinnamon - 2 teaspoons

• butter or hard margarine - 75 g (3 oz)

Instructions

• Preheat the oven to 190oC / Gas mark 5.

• Place the sliced apple in a small ovenproof pie dish and sprinkle with 25g / 1oz of the sugar. Mix the flour, oats, cinnamon and the remaining sugar together in a bowl.

• Cut up the butter or margarine into small pieces. Add the oats and rub in with your fingers until the mixture is crumbly.

• Sprinkle the crumble mixture evenly over the fruit.

• Bake for 40-50 minutes, until the crumble is golden brown and the fruit juices are bubbling up at the side.

• Serve with whipped cream if desired.

Nutrition Facts (Per Portion)

• Calories: 387kcal

• Carbohydrate: 58g

• Fat: 17g

- Protein: 5g

- Salt : 0.2g

- Sugar: 27g

- Potassium: 5.3mmol / 209mg

- Phosphate: 3.5 mmol / 110mg

CREAMY PORK CHOPS

Prep Time: 10 minutes

Cook Time: 20 minutes

Serving: 4

Ingredients

- pork chops - 450g / 18oz lean boneless

- onion - 1 medium (150g / 6oz) finely chopped

- vegetable oil - 1 tablespoon

- ginger - 1 – 2 teaspoons of powdered or minced, to taste

- double cream - 200mls / 6 ½ fluid ounces

Instructions

- Grill the pork chops

- Lightly brown onion in the vegetable oil. Add ginger to taste and cook for 1 minute with onion.

- Stir in cream and heat gently until sauce reduces a little.

- Pour over pork chop to serve.

Nutrition Facts (Per Portion)

- Calories: 601kcal

- Carbohydrate: 4g

- Fat: 55g

- Protein: 22g

- Salt : 0.2g

- Sugar: 3g

- Potassium: 398mg/ 10mmol

- Phosphate: 7.4mmol / 229mg

CORN AND CHEESE BALLS

Serving Size: 4 balls

Ingredients

- 2 cups frozen yellow corn

- 1 green chili

- 2 tablespoon cilantro

- 1/2 cup cottage cheese

- 4 slices white bread

- 1/2 cup all-purpose white flour

- 1 teaspoon chili powder

- 1 teaspoon cumin powder

- 1 teaspoon cilantro powder

- 1/4 teaspoon salt

- 2 cups vegetable oil

Preparation

- Thaw corn. Finely chop green chili and cilantro.

- In a mixing bowl, mix the cheese and thawed corn.

• Soak bread slices in water and squeeze out water so the bread becomes dry. Add this to corn and cheese mixture. Add flour, dry spices and cilantro. Mix it gently.

• Heat the oil in a large saucepan. Using a tablespoon, form small balls from the corn and cheese mixture and drop each ball into the hot oil. Cook until golden brown.

• Remove balls from the oil and place on a tray with kitchen napkin to drain excess oil.

• Serve hot with Cilantro Chutney.

Nutrients Facts Per Serving

• Calories 253

• Protein 7 g

• Carbohydrates 27 g

• Fat 13 g

• Cholesterol 3 mg

• Sodium 287 mg

• Potassium 169 mg

• Phosphorus 86 mg

• Calcium 46 mg

• Fiber 2.3 g

LAMB AND GINGER STIR FRY

Prep Time: 20 minutes

Cook Time: 10 minutes

Serving: 2

Ingredients

• lamb - 225g / 9oz, minced

• sunflower oil - 1 tablespoon

• fresh root ginger - 1 tablespoon, chopped or grated

• onion - 1 medium (150g / 6oz) chopped

• green pepper - 1 medium (150g / 6 oz) chopped

• red pepper - 1 medium (150g / 6 oz) chopped

• black pepper - 1 teaspoon, ground to taste

Instructions

• Fry the lamb at a high temperature in the sunflower oil for 3-4 minutes or until just browned.

• Add the root ginger, onion and peppers and fry for a further 2-3 minutes, stirring all the time.

• Season with pepper and serve.

Nutrition Facts (Per Portion)

- Calories: 336kcal
- Carbohydrate: 13g
- Fat: 21g
- Protein: 24g
- Salt : 0.2g
- Sugar: 11g
- Potassium: 18mmol / 710mg
- Phosphate: 9mmol / 272mg

Loaded Veggie Eggs

Prep Time: 5 minutes

Cook Time: 7 minutes

Total Time: 12-15 minutes

Yield: 2 servings

A versatile renal diet breakfast recipe to increase your intake of low potassium vegetables.

Ingredients

- 4 whole eggs
- 1 c cauliflower
- 3 c fresh spinach
- 1 garlic clove, minced

- 1/4 c bell pepper, chopped

- 1/4 cup onion, chopped

- 1/4 tsp black pepper

- 1 tbsp oil of choice (coconut or avocado oil is good for high heat)

- fresh parsley and spring onion for garnish

- optional tomatoes on side if no potassium restriction

Instructions

- Beat eggs with pepper until light and fluffy, set aside.

- Heat oil over medium heat in large skillet.

- Add onions and peppers to skillet and saute until peppers are translucent and golden.

- Add garlic, stirring quickly to combine and immediately adding cauliflower and spinach.

- Saute vegetables, turn heat to medium-low and cover for 5 minutes.

- Add eggs, stirring to combine with vegetables.

- When the eggs are cooked thoroughly, top with fresh parsley or spring onions. If no potassium restriction can serve with a side of bright fresh tomatoes topped with cracker black pepper. A touch of feta or a strong sharp cheese would also be delicious with these

Notes

- This is a great basic recipe for increasing your vegetable intake! Other spices/herbs that would be delicious with this include herbs de provence, red pepper flakes, extra garlic, and basil. I also like a little of lemon juice with my eggs to bring out the flavors rather than using salt.

• To reduce phosphorus further you can you 8 egg whites instead of egg yolks.

Nutrition Facts Serving Size: 1/2 recipe

• Calories Per Serving: 240

• Total Fat 16.6g

• Cholesterol 372mg

• Sodium 195mg

• Total Carbohydrate 7.8g

• Dietary Fiber 2.7g

• Protein 15.3g

• Vitamin A 389.2µg

• Vitamin C 54.6mg

• Iron 3.3mg

• Potassium 605.2mg

• Phosphorus 253.6mg

GRILLED CHICKEN PESTO PIZZA

Serving Size: 1/3rd pizza

Ingredients

• 1 Pizza Dough

• 1/2 cup orange bell pepper

• 1/2 cup yellow bell pepper

• 1/4 cup purple onion

• 1 tablespoon chives

• 2 tablespoons sun-dried tomato pesto

• 1 tablespoon olive oil

• 3/4 cup cooked chicken

• 1/3 cup grated Romano cheese

• 1/4 cup mozzarella cheese

• Olive oil for the grill

Instructions

• Dice the bell peppers, onion and chives. Chop or shred the chicken.

• Heat a tablespoon of olive oil and sauté the diced peppers and onion. Add the tomato pesto and cook for 2 minutes. Set aside for later.

• Roll or stretch the pizza dough to a 10-inch circle or rectangular shape. Set on a floured, rimless pizza sheet or sheet pan (unless you are using an oiled grill pizza pan). Let sit for about 5 minutes.

• Oil the grill surface and preheat the grill to hot heat.

• Put pizza dough on the grill (no toppings yet), and grill for about 2 to 3 minutes. Check bottom for browning; bubbles will form on top. Reduce to medium-high heat if needed to prevent burning. When light brown marks are visible on the bottom of the pizza dough, take the dough off the grill and place pizza dough with grill marks up.

• Top the pizza dough with the bell pepper, onion and pesto mixture. Top with the chicken, Romano cheese followed by the mozzarella cheese.

• Place the pizza back on the well-oiled grill or grill pan. Grill for another 2 to 3 minutes, until cheese is melted and the bottom of pizza is browned.

• Remove the pizza from the grill and garnish with chopped chives. Cut into 4 slices and serve.

Nutrients Facts Per Serving

• Calories 340

• Protein 21 g

• Carbohydrates 39 g

• Fat 18 g

• Cholesterol 46 mg

- Sodium 458 mg

- Potassium 375 mg

- Phosphorus 293 mg

- Calcium 204 mg

- Fiber 2.8 g

CINNAMON SUGAR COOKIES/DIALYSIS & KIDNEY FRIENDLY

Serves: 48 cookies/2 per serving

Ingredients

Cookie:

- 2-3/4 cups all-purpose flour

- 1-1/2 cups sugar (3/4 cup splenda sugar blend)

- 2 eggs

- 1 c butter, soft

- 1 teaspoon baking soda

- 2 teaspoon cream of tartar

- 1 1/4 teaspoons vanilla extract

To Roll In:

- 3 tablesppons sugar (3 tablespoons splenda sweetener)

- 1 1/2 teaspoons cinnamon

Instructions

- Put all the cookie ingredients in a large bowl and mix

together well.

• Mix the 3 tablespoons sugar and cinnamon together in a small bowl.

• Roll cookie dough into 1 inch balls and roll in the cinnamon and sugar mix.

• Put cookies on an ungreased cookie sheet about 2 inches apart and bake in a preheated 400 degree oven for about 8 to 10 minutes or until lightly browned.

ACORN SQUASH BAKED WITH PINEAPPLE

Serves: 2 servings

Ingredients

- 1 acorn squash, cut in half and seeded

- 2 teaspoons + 1 tablespoon unsalted butter

- 2 teaspoons brown sugar

- 3 tablespoons pineapple, crushed

- 1/4 teaspoon nutmeg

Preparation

- Preheat oven to 400 degrees.

- Place squash with cut side up in greased baking pan.

- Place one teaspoon butter plus one teaspoon brown sugar in each acorn half.

- Cover squash with aluminum foil and bake until tender, approximately 30 minutes.

- Scoop cooked squash out of shells, leaving 1/4 inch thick shell.

- Mix cooked squash, pineapple, 1 tablespoon butter, and nutmeg. Beat until smooth.

- Spoon mixture into shells; heat at 425 degrees for approximately 15 minutes.

Nutrition Facts Per Serving

- Calories 202

- Carbohydrates 31 g

- Protein 2 g

- Sodium 90 mg

- Potassium 783 mg

- Phosphorus 80 mg

ALASKA BAKED MACARONI AND CHEESE

Serves: 8 servings

Ingredients

- 3 cups elbow, small shell or bowtie pasta

- 2 tablespoons flour

- 2 tablespoons unsalted butter

- 2 cups milk

- 1 teaspoon mustard powder

- 1 teaspoon paprika

- 1 tablespoon fresh thyme or tarragon, chopped or 1 teaspoon dry

- 2 cups cheese (gouda, cheddar, or any combo)

- croutons or chopped almonds to taste

Preparation

- Heat oven to 350 degrees.

- Boil pasta in a large pot until al-dente.

• Meanwhile, in a medium glass measuring cup, measure flour and butter. Microwave about 1-2 minutes until golden brown.

• Slowly stir in milk and continue microwaving until thickened. Stir in spices and herbs.

• Mix drained noodles, sauce, and cheese and put in a greased casserole dish. Bake about 20 minutes.

• Top with croutons or chopped almonds in the last 5 minutes.

Nutrition Facts Per Serving

• Calories 424

• Carbohydrates 36 g

• Protein 22 g

• Dietary Fiber 2g

• Fat 20g

• Sodium 479 mg

• Potassium 237 mg

• Phosphorus 428 mg

Maple Pancakes

Serving Size: 2-4 pancakes

Ingredients

• 1 cup all-purpose flour

• 1 tablespoon granulated sugar

- 2 teaspoons baking powder

- 1/8 teaspoon salt

- 2 large egg whites

- 1 cup 1% low-fat milk

- 2 tablespoons canola oil

- 1 tablespoon maple extract

Instructions

- In a medium mixing bowl combine the flour, sugar, baking powder and salt. Make a well in the center of the dry mixture. Set aside.

- In a large mixing bowl combine the egg whites, milk, oil and maple extract.

- Add egg mixture all at once into to the dry mixture. Stir just until moistened (batter should be lumpy).

- To make 4" pancakes, pour about 1/4 cup batter onto a hot, lightly greased griddle or heavy skillet.

- Cook over medium heat about 2 minutes on each side or until pancakes are golden. Flip the pancake when it has bubbly surface and edges are slightly dry. To keep pancakes light and fluffy, turn only once and avoid pressing with the spatula.

Nutrients Facts Per Serving

- Calories 178

- Protein 6 g

- Carbohydrates 25 g

- Fat 6 g

- Cholesterol 2 mg
- Sodium 297 mg
- Potassium 126 mg
- Phosphorus 116 mg
- Calcium 174 mg
- Fiber 0.7 g

APPLE & CHERRY CHUTNEY

Ingredients

- 1 medium tart apple

- 1 cup dried tart cherries

- 1 small red onion, thinly sliced

- 1 cup apple cider vinegar

- 1 1/2 cups sugar

Preparation

- Quarter and core the apple and cut into thin slices, leaving the skin on.

- Put the apples and cherries in a heavy saucepan with the onions, vinegar, and sugar. Cook, stirring until the sugar is dissolved and the mixture is beginning to boil.

- Cover and reduce heat to low and cook until the onions are tender and the dried cherries are plump and tender, about 8-10 minutes.

- Uncover and bring the heat up to high and boil until the syrup around the fruit is reduced to a shiny glaze, about 5 minutes more. Chutney may be served at once or kept, covered and refrigerated for several days.

Nutrition Facts Per Serving

- Calories 55
- Carbohydrates 14 g
- Protein 1 g
- Sodium 2 mg
- Potassium 12 mg
- Phosphorus 1 mg

Apple Filled Crepes

Ingredients

- 4 egg yolks
- 2 whole eggs
- 1/2 cup sugar
- 1 cup flour
- 1/4 cup oil
- 2 cups milk
- 4 apples
- 1/2 cup brown sugar
- 1/2 teaspoon cinnamon
- 1/2 teaspoon nutmeg
- 1 stick or 1/2 cup unsalted butter

Preparation

- Mix egg yolks, whole eggs, sugar, flour, oil, and milk until the batter is free of lumps.

- Heat a small non-stick skillet over medium heat.

- Spray pan with cooking spray.

- Using a 2 ounce ladle or 1/4 cup, spoon 1 scoop of batter into the pan, then swirl the pan to spread the crepe batter thinly on the bottom of the pan.

- Cook for about 20 seconds, then flip the crepe (with the aid of a rubber spatula) and cook for about 10 seconds. Set crepes aside while you make the filling.

- Peel, core, and slice apples each into 12 slices.

- Heat a medium saute pan.

- Melt butter, then add brown sugar.

- Toss in the apples, cinnamon, and nutmeg.

- Cook apples until tender but not mushy. Set aside to cool.

Assembling the Crepes:

- Fill the middle of each crepe about with about 2 tablespoons of apple filling.

- Roll into a log.

Note

- Crepes can be made the day before or hours in advance, just cover with plastic wrap and store in the refrigerator. When ready to eat microwave crepes for a few seconds.

Nutrition Facts Per Serving

- Calories 315
- Carbohydrates 40 g
- Protein 5 g
- Dietary Fiber 15 g
- Sodium 356 mg
- Potassium 160 mg
- Phosphorus 103 mg